# Decoding the Enigma: His Guide to Her Menopause

# Decoding the Enigma: His Guide to Her Menopause

Robert M. Chell, Ph.D.
Jane Cooper, MA

iUniverse, Inc.
New York  Lincoln  Shanghai

**Decoding the Enigma: His Guide to Her Menopause**

iUniverse books may be ordered through booksellers or by contacting:

iUniverse
2021 Pine Lake Road, Suite 100
Lincoln, NE 68512
www.iuniverse.com
1-800-Authors (1-800-288-4677)

ISBN-13: 978-0-595-38971-1 (pbk)
ISBN-13: 978-0-595-83354-2 (ebk)
ISBN-10: 0-595-38971-6 (pbk)
ISBN-10: 0-595-83354-3 (ebk)

Printed in the United States of America

This book is dedicated to our spouses, Beverly and Donald, whose support and encouragement throughout the writing of this book have been immeasurable.

# ACKNOWLEDGEMENTS

This book has profited from the experiences of many individuals. In particular those who participated in our focus groups and whose life experiences and wisdom we incorporated into this guide.

We wish to give special thanks to Dr. Lona Whitmarsh, colleague and friend, who made many significant contributions during the initial stages of the writing process.

In addition, a major thank you to our spouses, Beverly and Donald, who were so instrumental in the advising and editing functions associated with this book.

# TABLE OF CONTENTS

# INTRODUCTION

He says: "Did I do something wrong?"
She says: "No!"
He says: "Why are you so upset?"
She says: "I don't want to talk about it."
He says: "There must be something wrong."
She says: "Nothing's wrong."
He says: "Then what's the problem?"
She says: "You just don't understood."

Does this dialogue sound familiar? Is this similar to a conversation that you have had with the woman in your life? If so, she may be one of the millions of women who is nearing the age of 55.

What makes 55 the typical age to be having this type of discussion? The answer is: That's the most common age for women to go through menopause. Conversations like this are only one of the many issues that you and she may be dealing with as a result of menopause.

What is menopause, who is this menopausal woman, how long does this menopause "thing" last, and very importantly, how are the results of menopause going to affect you?

The answers lie in the following pages. However, just as you are asking these questions, she may be thinking things like:

- I see my mother when I look in the mirror.
- I'm angry, but I don't know why.
- I'm reminiscing too much about things that happened years ago.
- I look at younger people and am envious of their appearance and energy level.

- I'm having a hard time remembering things and it frightens me.
- I feel sad and tearful for no apparent reason.
- I'm always sapped of energy and do not know why.
- I can't sleep yet I am so tired.
- I'm afraid that my friends, co-workers, and family are changing the way they think of me.

Believe it or not, menopause is not just the province of the aging matron. These kinds of questions may be raised by women who are only in their mid 30's and who may be transitioning into the process of menopause. "Menopause?" you say, "Not her. She's too young!"

Guess what? If she is experiencing these symptoms, she is not too young. The process of menopause can last for a number of years before the female body actually transitions to the stage when a woman no longer has her monthly period. The woman in your life may not be going crazy or experiencing early senile dementia or becoming an insomniac, she may simply be experiencing the beginning of a long hormonally based process.

There are many myths about menopause, and you and she must recognize that they are just that—MYTHS. One of them is that menopause is a change that occurs within a couple of years. Not true. Menopause occurs in three stages; it begins with perimenopause, which can start as early as in a woman's 30s, followed by menopause, which is when menstrual periods cease for an entire calendar year, ending with postmenopause, sometimes lasting for another five years. The menopausal process may take 10 years or longer.

*Decoding the Enigma: His Guide to Her Menopause* is written to help you understand the recent changes in thought associated with the menopausal process. Women in the past have suffered as a result of many misconceptions that are due to the lack of adequate communication about menopausal issues. There is a body of old wives' tales that seem to have been perpetuated from one generation to another. A major purpose of this book is to dispel these myths and to give men constructive strategies to cope with menopause.

The menopausal woman may notice some psychological as well physical differences that concern her while she is experiencing menopause. However, every woman does not experience menopause in the same way. For that reason her personal "Life Strategy Orientation" (**LSO**) becomes an important variable in helping you and her through perimenopause, menopause, and postmenopause. Her **LSO** is the way she interacts with the people in her life, gathers information about her world and makes decisions about life events. Her transition through the menopausal years will be different from her mother's. This is NOT her mother's menopause.

## WHAT IS THIS "THING" CALLED MENOPAUSE?

Our mothers' generation defined menopause as the end of menstruation. We know differently. What we typically label as menopausal behavior begins with perimenopause. This stage can begin even earlier than age 35, long before the cessation of menstruation. During this period, the hormones surge and fluctuate. Many women who are logical and rational in most spheres of their lives find that during this stage their thoughts are confused, and their emotions are in full flight.

## WHO IS THIS MENOPAUSAL WOMAN?

Once a woman reaches this stage, what "changes" can she expect to encounter over the next 15 to 20 years? The female hormones (estrogen and progesterone) will gradually become depleted, and as this happens, a woman's emotional and psychological behavior may be affected. Some women have barely any physical or psychological symptoms, while others experience noticeable differences that impact their life decisions and long-term relationships. This latter group of women will likely experience a wide range of conflicting emotions and behaviors that they have never experienced before, making them strangers to friends and even to themselves.

## DOES MENOPAUSE HAVE TO SPELL "WITCH?"

Much of menopausal behavior is hormonally driven, creating a situation where emotions override the intellect. Men's responses to menopause may also be emotional, since they may be confronting behavior that they have never seen before, coming from someone whom they thought they knew well. How is it possible for a woman who may have successfully managed a household, raised children, and/or achieved responsible positions in an organization to become easily threatened and overly emotional? The answer may not lie only in her fluctuating hormones but where she is in her *hierarchy of needs*. The hierarchy of needs, based on one of the most famous theories of motivation, was developed by Abraham Maslow[1].

This may seem academic, and at this point you may be saying to yourself, is this going to be a lecture? Hang in there, this is important information and may help you understand what may be happening psychologically to the menopausal woman in your life.

What is a hierarchy of needs? Our most basic needs, which sit at the bottom of the hierarchy, are for physiological survival and security. These needs are for such things as air, water, food, sleep, sex, the security of a home and a family. If our needs for survival and security are not satisfied, our focus will be upon their satisfaction. For example, if you are in the desert without water your focus will be upon getting water. Until this need is satisfied, seeking water will dominate your behavior.

Once the basic needs are satisfied we can then move on to the next level of the hierarchy, which includes the social and esteem needs such as love and the need to belong, to be accepted by others, to be respected and to be seen as competent by others. The highest level in the hierarchy of needs is self-actualization, which is frequently defined as *achieving one's fullest potential*. Reaching the self-actualization level is a life-long process.

Are you curious as to why this is relevant to a discussion about menopause? In addition to the physiological symptoms a woman may experience during menopause (hot flashes, loss of energy, muscle aches and pains), she may also experience difficulty in concentration, problem solving and memory. Her sense of competency, and consequently her sense of security, may be threatened. When this happens, once again she becomes focused upon satisfying her security needs. Just as one can go up the hier-

---

[1] Maslow, A.H, (1954). *Motivation and personality.* New York: Harper & Row

archy of needs, one can go down the hierarchy of needs. Is it any wonder that her decreased feelings of competency make her feel insecure, overly sensitive and easily threatened?

Here's a situation that illustrates the concept of needs: You have occupied a position in an organization that has provided you with a great deal of satisfaction regarding your social and esteem needs (you have received promotions, are part of the bowling team, have a regular group for lunch). As a result of reaching this level in the needs hierarchy, you may be close to self-actualization (the "be all that you can be" stage). Then your boss calls you in on Friday (and it usually is on a Friday), and tells you that your services are no longer needed. Are you concerned with self-actualization now? Of course not! You are more concerned with how you will pay your mortgage or your MasterCard bill. Your survival and security needs will now dominate your behavior.

## WHAT TO EXPECT

Just as we are all complex 'beings' with different needs at different times in our lives, we also have individual personality temperaments. Throughout this guide we will present you with an opportunity to "figure out" the personality temperament of the menopausal woman in your life and identify her Life Strategy Orientation (**LSO**). We present specific and general coping strategies — specific to a woman's temperament and general to all menopausal women. Men will become educated regarding their specific roles in this process, and what strategies they need to implement to ease her through this "change." Additionally, you will also learn how to help make this a smooth transition.

## IS THIS GOING TO BE OVER SOON AND WITH WHAT RESULT?

Menopause, euphemistically referred to as "The Change", is a process that can last from six to thirteen years. You will find "The Change" to be an extraordinary challenge to you and your relationship with the menopausal woman. The purpose of this guide is to help you not only survive this process but to also gain knowledge and the strategies to help your relationship **thrive** during this stage and beyond. We make the distinction between surviving the process (muddling through it to the end) and thriving (making lemonade out of lemons), thus affording you the opportunity to grow and develop in your relationship. Many long-term relationships become habit with habitual ways of behaving and communicating. Too much of how we act and react is predictable and comfortable. As a result, our behaviors often become static and stagnant, and we do not feel fully satisfied. People often say, "well, maybe that's all there is." Well maybe that is NOT all there is. Menopause can be the instigator of positive change; change for the better. You and she can learn new ways to problem-solve and relate to each other as a couple.

To **thrive** you need to:

- See this stage as an opportunity for positive changes in your relationship

- Introduce into your relationship new strategies and techniques that we suggest in this book

- Become more knowledgeable about menopause's physiological and psychological effects

- Gain more understanding of the behaviors that may be a result of menopause

- Develop greater empathy for the challenges that she will face during menopause

## IS THIS PROCESS GOING TO BE CHALLENGING?

**OF COURSE.** Going through the process with her may at times be tough. Oftentimes you may feel as though you have reached a "fork in the road." One direction may be to walk away emotionally and physically, becoming less involved in the relationship, spending more time at work, on the golf course, in a bar. This is not unusual. Recent marriage statistics reveal an astonishing fact: There has been a dramatic increase in the number of separations leading to divorce after 20, 30 or more years of marriage[2]. Menopause may be one cause.

---

[2] *A House Divided* by Elizabeth Enright. www.aarpmagazine.org/family/articles/a2004-05-26-mg-divorce.html

The other direction is to opt to make the relationship **thrive**. What is the necessary ingredient? Motivation. Why should you be motivated? So that you can experience the joy that comes from sharing and expanding the depth of your relationship.

If you are motivated, how do you develop the knowledge, understanding and empathy to see her through this life transition? The answer to these questions is…read further.

**The contents of this book will:**
- Introduce the A, B, C to Z's of menopause
- Identify the menopausal woman's orientation to her world and the people in it
- Help the man understand her Life Strategy Orientation (**LSO**)
- Recognize challenges unique to her experience of menopause
- Provide the man with creative action plans to enhance the relationship

**Let's start!**

# CHAPTER ONE

# WHAT DID I DO? PROBABLY NOTHING! WHAT SHOULD YOU DO?

She says:    "The temperature in this pool is just too cold."
He says:     "I don't think 82 degrees is too cold. A pool that is too warm is just not refreshing."
She says:    "Why do you only think about yourself? Isn't it important to you that I think it's too cold?"
He says:     "When did I become responsible for the temperature of the pool?"
She says:    "With all I do around the house, that's the least you can do."
He says:     "You're the one who wanted the pool in the first place and no matter what temperature I make the pool it won't be right."
She says:    "There you go again, always blaming me when you know you're wrong."

Does this conversation sound logical and rational? How do mundane conversations like this devolve into a battleground between two normally rational people?

Men and women will often interpret conversations quite differently from each other, and situations like the one above can be exacerbated by menopause. How often have you been surprised by the fact that you were in the **same** room for the **same** conversation but walked away with a totally **different** picture of what was said? We ask that you look at these and similar situations from not only your vantage point, but hers as well.

1

We ask that you "step into her shoes," and sensitize yourself to the mis-communications and misunderstandings that so often get in the way.

**From his shoes she has changed:**
- From predictable to unpredictable
- From high-energy level to low-energy level
- From certain to uncertain
- From independent to dependent
- From thoughtful to forgetful
- From even-tempered to short-fused
- From concerned about others to overly concerned about herself

**From her shoes she has changed:**
- From feeling in control to feeling overwhelmed
- From feeling secure to feeling insecure
- From feeling invincible to feeling vulnerable
- From feeling attractive to feeling unattractive
- From being emotional to being overly emotional
- From being tolerant to being irritable

As you can see, the psychological effects are often far greater than the physiological changes that occur. Indeed, if you only had to deal with the physiological changes you might find it far easier to cope with her menopause (after all, don't they have pills for this?). Physiology is a science. Science is logical and rational. Men prefer logic and rationality. Therefore, when a problem exists, you seek a rational, logical solution, one that is workable and practical. Dealing with a menopausal woman requires more than that. Indeed, very often she does not want your solution, only your understanding.

Men, who have solved problems ranging from a nuclear energy crisis to an annoying rattle in an automobile engine, are baffled by the behavioral changes they encounter in menopausal women. Suddenly, questions such as, do I look old, do I look fat, and do I look like my mother are being asked with greater frequency. Do you know the right answers to these questions? Are you asking yourself (and within yourself the question must stay), "If she owns a mirror, why is she asking me these questions?" Are you afraid to answer these questions? Do you feel that whatever you say will be wrong? Even when you give what you feel is the optimal answer, you may not have necessarily solved the problem. Remember, depending on the situation the optimal answer may not always be the truest answer. It is confusing to figure out why she is asking these questions and what she really wants from you.

What she is really saying is:

- "Am I still attractive?"
- "Am I still loveable?"
- "Am I still everything I was 20 years ago?"

Menopause frequently threatens a woman's self-concept, her sense of personal worth. In our society, which emphasizes youth and physical attractiveness and undervalues the aging process, menopause is a signal that her youth is over and she has transitioned to middle age. This is a critical time when a woman feels vulnerable and experiences a strong need to be needed.

You need to affirm in her mind that she is still attractive, still lovable and still worthwhile. Let her know that she continues to meet your expectations and that you still value her. It is necessary to **listen** to the meaning behind her words and not take them at face value. At this point, she is hoping for affirmation and understanding. Since this is an emotional need, your words and actions must often be repeated. It is not like a statement of a fact, which only requires one presentation. Each of us needs to be told and shown that we are loved on a consistent basis. We do not find it satisfying when someone says: "You know I told you I loved you a month ago. Nothing has changed." Each of us requires this continual kind of affirmation to satisfy our emotional needs.

As a man you are not immune to this emotional need for affirmation and understanding. Changes are happening to you too. Change happens to all of us. By "standing in her shoes" it will be easier for you to develop a perspective of a situation from her vantage point. All that may be required is a simple comment such as "I understand." What is also important is that you control yourself and hold back from making critical remarks when she does present the questions you believe are ridiculous and even childlike.

## ARE YOU TELLING ME THIS IS A FAILURE TO COMMUNICATE?

To develop a good relationship between you and the menopausal woman, communication is essential. Communication has become a hackneyed phrase that is often viewed as the panacea for all relationship problems. However, in this particular situation, the nature of communication is critical. The "receiver" needs to provide the "sender" with feedback that the intended message has been understood. This might be a verbal response such as "yes, dear," "mmm, hmm," or even a nod of the head. Many believe that without undivided attention it is not possible to listen. How often have you heard the phrase "If you are not looking at me, how can you be listening?" There is an important distinction between hearing and listening. Hearing is the sense by which sound is perceived. Listening involves an interpretation of what has been said and giving appropriate feedback. How is appropriateness determined? Appropriateness depends on our intentions. Intentions might be...

- Do you want her to know that you understood the message?
- Do you want her to know that you agree with the message?
- Do you want her to hear from you what she wants to hear?
- Do you want her to hear from you what she needs to hear?

How often do you hear her say, "You're not listening" or "You don't understand"?

Let's look at an example.

The setting: You are watching an NFL playoff game. You are comfortably seated in your favorite recliner with your favorite snack food and liquid refreshment. Your team is at the five-yard line and the quarterback is ready to throw the winning touchdown pass. She comes into the room.

She says: "Should I cook dinner or should we order a pizza?"

He says: "Whatever you want."

She says: "Why are the food decisions always left up to me?"

He says: "*!*!*!*!"

She says: "Why are you getting so angry at me?"

He says: "My team just blew a touchdown"

She says: "Did you hear a word I said? As usual, you aren't paying any attention to me."

He says: "All I really want to do is relax and watch a lousy game of football. Is that too much to ask?"

She says: "And all I really want is for you to pay attention to me instead of the television."

Have you had this conversation? Does this sound familiar? This kind of dialogue is one you probably have had many times before at different times in your life. However, her sensitivities tend to be heightened during menopause. How did one innocuous question escalate into a conflict? Before menopause you and your partner probably let interactions like this one roll off your back. However, during menopause, minor issues often trigger unspoken anger, frustration, stress and anxiety. This is caused by a lack of understanding of each other's needs and expectations. Consider this perspective:

**His shoes:** I have been working to support this family. I go out there eight to ten hours a day and often have my brains bashed in! I take abuse, "Yes, boss, anything you say, boss". "The customer is always right". "I'll get that delivery to you as soon as possible." There never seems to be enough money. I get little time for myself. She needs. The kids need. My needs come last.

**Her shoes:** For years I put the needs of my family above my own, worried about finances, provided a safe and healthy environment for my family, worked within a limited budget, never felt appreciated, not only by my family but also by the outside world. I didn't need a paycheck to feel appreciated; just your letting me know that I'm important.

It is obvious that there is a history of pent up feelings underlying the innocent dialogue between these two parties. Yes, these feelings do occur throughout a relationship, however, during menopause they are felt with greater intensity.

Another communication debacle occurs when you listen to the words of her message, but you just do not understand the underlying meaning of her words. Does the following situation sound familiar?

| | |
|---|---|
| He says: | "Hon, your birthday is coming up, what would you like?" |
| She says: | "I can't think of anything. Oh, I don't really need anything." |
| He says: | "Are you sure?" |
| She says: | "I don't want you to bother, it's ok." |
| He says: | "If you think of anything, let me know" |

Her birthday arrives and you celebrate it with a lovely birthday card and a big hug and kiss. Days later...

| | |
|---|---|
| He says: | "You've been acting differently. What's the matter?" |
| She says: | "Don't you know?" |
| He says: | "Know what?" |
| She says: | "I can't believe you didn't get me anything for my birthday." |
| He says: | "I asked you what you wanted and you said you didn't want anything. Didn't you say that?" |
| She says: | "I guess you just don't understand." |

You will walk away feeling confused and frustrated. Remember, women who are accustomed to satisfying others' needs before their own are reluctant to ask for things for themselves. After all, you did exactly what she asked you to do, but you were still wrong. Do you want to know how to win points with her? Learn what kinds of gifts she likes and buy them for her even when she says: "I don't want anything." Learn to listen, not just to hear.

It sounds like a cliché, but support and supportive communication are important. Supportive communication involves affirmation of the woman and recognition of how difficult this process may be for her. Because you are an action-oriented individual, your first response is to want to change the menopausal process. But you cannot. What you can do is provide support and supportive communication. During menopause women experience a strong sense of vulnerability and insecurity. She looks to you for words and behaviors that remind her that she is still desirable, attractive and important in your life. She is hoping for timely reminders of your affection. Gift-giving is an important behavior that shows your thoughtfulness, caring and her continued worth in your life. The gifts are merely symbols that you think about her, and she is a priority in your life. These words and behaviors are an affirmation of your concern during this difficult period in her life.

## TO REACT OR NOT TO REACT—
## THAT IS THE QUESTION!

At times, you will be tempted to ignore the situation because you have no rational, logical, workable solution to deal with what is taking place. Your inaction often triggers emotional responses of anger and frustration. You sense that she expects you to do something, but what is that something? Historically, men have been the hunters. Hunters see the goal and establish a strategy to achieve it. Men still see themselves in the modern manifestations of this role. In most aspects of your life, as a man, you are expected to take action and achieve a result. However, what is it that you are expected to do in this case? Once you have established the menopausal woman's **LSO**, you will have the answer.

## OLD WIVES' AND OLD HUSBANDS' TALES

One of the things that has made menopause such an enigma until recently is that there was little direct dialogue about *"the Change,"* also referred to as the "secret affliction," or "middle age crazy." When there was communication, it occurred in hushed tones, and a great deal of this communication tended to be miscommunication, much of which was shared from generation to generation, from women to women or men to men, in the form of "old wives tales." Rarely was there direct communication between the sexes regarding menopause. Many were reluctant to acknowledge that menopause was actually taking place. Furthermore, it might have been viewed as an impolite topic of conversation. As a way of learning more about menopause, how about trying the following quiz, which will help you separate fact from fiction.

- Menopause is a short stage in life that only affects women in their 50's.
  **True      False**

False. This is a three-stage process that may begin when a woman is in her early to mid 40's and may last well into her 50's. These stages will be discussed in the A to Z's of menopause.

- All women going through menopause lose interest in sex.
  **True      False**

False. At least 50% of menopausal women report no change in sexual interest. Only 20% notice any marked lack of interest. According to the American Association of Retired Persons, you and your partner may find yourselves enjoying your sex life now more than ever. Why? You share less concern about pregnancy, and with the the maturing of your children, time that has been consumed by active parenting responsibilities is now available as leisure time for both of you.

- All women going through menopause lose their memory and thinking skills.
  **True      False**

False. Women have no greater loss of cognitive functioning than men.

- All women going through *the Change* become depressed
  **True      False**

False. The American College of Obstetricians and Gynecologists report that rates of depression are actually higher among women of childbearing age.

- Women under the age of 45 are too young to be experiencing menopausal symptoms.
  **True**    **False**

False. Menopausal symptoms may begin as early as a woman's mid 30s.

Be honest, how many did you answer correctly? If you did not answer many correctly, you are part of the majority. Even though menopause has become a topic of conversation and receives a significant amount of media attention, a great at deal of misinformation is still communicated. How can you discern what is good information and what is not? In order to survive and thrive during your partner's menopausal years, we will "decode" for you the kind of information you need to know and provide strategies to deal with specific everyday situations.

## HEART VS MIND

It is important to be proactive. Too often what complicates our understanding of the issues related to menopause is that we address them in a reactive rather than proactive fashion. As a result, the reaction is emotional rather than intellectual.

The setting: The husband arrives home from work and finds his wife lying on the couch crying.

He says: "What's wrong? Are you ok?"

She says: "I don't know what's wrong with me. About an hour ago I had this weird feeling and started sweating to the point where my clothes were drenched, and I lost every ounce of energy."

He says: "Maybe you should call the doctor."

She says: "No, I feel better now, just drained. I'm embarrassed because everyone at work saw me drenched."

He says: "Are you sure we shouldn't call the doctor?"

This could become a very emotional and tense discussion. When we are feeling frightened and concerned, these emotions cause our perceptions to become clouded. It is useful to anticipate situations before they occur so that they can be better managed clearly, objectively and unemotionally. If, for example, the husband in this case knew the physical and psychological effects of menopause, rather than suggesting that his wife rush to call the doctor, he would have understood that "hot flashes" are a normal symptom of menopause.

We will be providing you with a series of actions, reactions and concepts that should help you become proactive and react more effectively to the menopausal woman in your life.

## SHE'S NOT CHANGING, SHE'S EVOLVING

Menopause is an evolutionary process. There are many benefits associated with this time. It may be the first time in her life when a woman can begin to focus upon herself. Although other life events may compete with this focus, there is increased time for her to think about her needs and desires. Many women report, for example, that it is much better to be a grandparent than a parent. You can enjoy the fun times and you can return the grandchildren to their parents when they become cranky. This is also a time that may be associated with increased economic freedom and the opportunity for her to return to school, re-enter the workforce, or fully focus on a career. The major family expenses are over and the money that was targeted for the benefit of others can now be spent on husband and wife. Now is the time to get the car that you have always wanted or to take your dream trip. If you listen to the television commercial, you can even to go to Disney World without the children. You can begin to recognize that it is truly your turn, and the best is yet to come.

## IS CHANGE BAD?

There is a natural tendency for men to ignore the psychological changes that are occurring as a result of menopause and deny their existence. You may look for ways to escape this situation. What do you think are the most common routes?

- the golf course
- the local bar
- the office

It might surprise you to find that "the office" is the most common escape route. This is called "escape into reality." You busy yourself with so many work tasks that you are able to avoid the situation with no guilt attached. No one can fault you for working extra hours, whereas they could if you were engaging in leisure activities. After all, who would choose work over the golf course? You avoid the situation in a socially acceptable manner by focusing upon career or civic responsibilities.

It is also possible to "escape" without leaving home. Do you hide behind the newspaper, television program, food, drugs, alcohol or sleep? How many of those "escapes" apply to you? Recognize that any of these strategies are temporary fixes; the issues and problems still remain. Escape from the situation is also possible by hanging out with a crowd of friends. There is "safety in numbers" because people typically do not discuss their problems in front of others. Keeping the social calendar crammed is another way of avoiding being alone with her. Beware of the "ostrich effect." Not addressing the problem does not make it disappear.

This is your guide to her menopause, and therefore it is appropriate that as a guide it is directed to your understanding and your actions regarding the menopausal process. We are not asking that you become a candidate for sainthood, however some situations require "saint-like" actions. Recognize that satisfying her needs does not preclude you from satisfying your own needs. As we have stated before, you have a lot invested in this relationship, and you want to continue happily. There are going to be a number of situations that will frustrate you and make you angry, even though you know the underlying cause is menopausal. However, knowing the underlying cause of the behavior does not soften the negativity of the behavior. Consider the following:

She says:    "I needed to call you at work and get you out of your meet-
             ing because they only delivered half of the furniture we
             ordered.
             You need to call the store and remedy the situation."
He says:     "Why did you get me out of this meeting, can't you call the
             store yourself?"
She says:    "You know you'll get better results, they listen to men bet-
             ter than they listen to women."
He says:     "All right, all right, I'll take care of it."

Later that evening…

She says:    "We still didn't get the furniture that we were promised."
He says:     "I spoke with the manager and he promised it would be
             delivered."
She says:    "Are you sure you spoke to the right manager? You know
             you don't pay attention to detail the way I do."
He says:     "If you thought you could do a better job, then why didn't
             you do it?"
She says:    "Maybe I should have."

Are you angry yet? Anger is provoked by constraints. What do you do
with the anger? It is important to address the anger that you may feel during this period. A common strategy that is employed in situations like this
one is that of "swallowing the anger." This means not articulating or vent-
ing the anger that you feel. Swallowing the anger avoids confrontation.
You may both do this because of a basic fear of confrontation. You fear
confrontation because you feel it will put your relationship at risk. In
truth, the lack of confrontation is riskier. Anger that is not expressed smol-
ders into hostility. Hostility, in turn, causes a growing wedge in your relationship.

Another by-product of anger and hostility is aggression. Aggression is
defined as a desire to hurt or injure another person or thing physically or
verbally. The first reaction to aggression is to react in kind. Which of the
following best describes your actions? Do you:

- hit back?
- punch a wall?
- throw an object?
- shout expletives?
- say something nasty and cutting?

You must understand that revenge only exacerbates the situation and further intensifies the sense of aggression. What are the consequences of your actions? What are the results you want to achieve? Remember, do not act out of anger. Think strategically. The old maxim regarding "winning battles and losing wars" becomes operative here. What does this maxim mean? Although we may triumph in a particular incident, the overall effect of our actions can damage our long-term relationship.

The setting: You have planned a 25th anniversary dinner at her favorite restaurant and you have shopped for a special gift to mark the occasion.

He says: "After 25 years together this is a token of my affection."

She says: "Oh, this is nice," with a lack of enthusiasm.

He says: "Don't you like it?"

She says: "It's very nice but I'm not sure I will be able to wear it that much."

He says: "If you don't like it, I'll take it back."

She says: "No, no, I'll keep it.

He says: "Don't do me any favors; I feel that I can never win with you."

What has happened in this scenario? Obviously, he is angry at what he perceives to be her lack of appreciation. He did not get what he expected in terms of her appreciation; he is disappointed and frustrated. As we stated before, frustration leads to aggression. As a result, he responds by giving her a "zinger." He has succeeded in winning "the battle". He feels bad now that she feels bad. But what effect does this have on the supposed celebration and what long-term impact does it have on the relationship? Perhaps "the war" has been lost. In subsequent chapters we will discuss appropriate strategies; be prepared to channel your anger and control your aggression!

## WHAT CAN YOU DO?

What should be done? Who should be involved? You can do a lot and you can be involved. How women respond to menopause is similar to how they have dealt with other life issues. There are a great many individual differences in the way menopause is experienced. Not only are there individual differences in physiological reactions and symptoms, but also in the psychological and behavioral reactions that take place. How women respond to menopause is often a function of how they have dealt with other life issues. Many life issues require problem-solving strategies. We call these approaches "Life Strategy Orientations" (LSOs). These LSOs are a key predictor of her psychological and behavioral reactions to menopause. You are provided in Chapter Three with a short questionnaire that will enable you to identify the LSOs of the woman in your life. As we have pointed out, menopause is not experienced in isolation; you need to develop effective coping strategies (co-strategies). Different LSOs require different co-strategies; in other words, joint and shared techniques for both of you to employ. How nice and simple it would be if it could be said that all you need to do is implement a 5-step co-strategy. It is not that simple. However, there are certain general co-strategies that are effective regardless of a woman's LSO. In later chapters we offer both specific co-strategies (for the LSO of your wife) and general strategies to all women experiencing menopausal changes.

# CHAPTER TWO

# THE A TO Z OF MENOPAUSE: DECODING THE ENIGMA

Each woman lives through the menopausal process differently. It would be helpful to be able to look through a crystal ball that will predict menopausal symptoms, but that is not likely. Many of us only know about menopause through the eyes of others. Moreover, many of us think that the transition to menopause will have more negatives than positives. Why? When menopause is discussed, it is usually the negatives that are stressed. What you will find in this chapter are many of the "positives" associated with the menopausal process. However, just reading through our A to Z may not be enough. Share them with your partner and remind her, when she is feeling low, that there are at least 26 reasons for her to feel good about this stage of her life. Become her "menopause coach" and, in the tradition of coaching, serve as her private tutor and her valuable support system.

It is also important to recognize that many of these "positives" may come and go. Remember that menopause is a process and patience is necessary. Although you may view this section as an attempt to make lemonade out of lemons, remember that these "positives" are real, taken from personal experiences and focus groups, to help you become her "A-rated" coach.

**Acceptance:** Menopause is a process, one that all women experience whether by age or surgery. Finding the best action plan[3] to deal with it and

---

[3] Action plan: state the goal you want to achieve and then establish a strategy to achieve that goal. It should include short-range, concrete and challenging objectives, which serve as a pathway to achieving the goal.

taking an active versus a passive approach, will enable you and your partner to be aware of all the possibilities. Accept and embrace the change!

**Benefits**: You and she know yourselves better at this stage of life than at any previous time. The result is that you both can be aware of your needs and place priority upon satisfying them. Up to this point she, in particular, has been concerned with other's needs before her own. Perhaps you have both been nurturing children, building careers, or planning for the future. The future is now! It is your turn to really start enjoying the freedom this stage of life brings.

**Caring**: There will be increased opportunities for caring for one's self as well as others. She can spend more time focusing on herself and what she needs and wants to accomplish. Has she put off that gym membership, daily walk, week at the spa or those long luxurious baths?

**Development**: This is a wonderful opportunity for her to think in terms of personal, educational and career development. Does she want to go back to school? Does she want to start a small business? Does she want to start reading the books that have been sitting on her bookshelf?

**Evolving**: Remind her that this is the next chapter in her life. As she transitions into this phase, guide her toward focusing on the positive changes that she can look forward to. There is no reason for her to resist or fear change. She can be **at least** as successful in the future as she was in the past.

**Follow-through**: Direct her toward persevering with her action-plan and not getting off-track. Now is the time for her to concentrate on herself and her needs. If, by chance, she does get off-track, remind her that it is all right. As Scarlett O'Hara said, "Tomorrow is another day."

**Growth**: Whether she has set personal growth, career growth or financial growth goals, it is important that she actually write them down, along with an action plan. Make certain she asks herself and finds the answers to questions like: Why and for whom is growth necessary? Ask her what particular needs will be satisfied when she achieves her goals and how important the satisfaction of those needs are to her. Help her to assess what she wants versus what she needs.

**Harmony:** Concentrate on what is good and eliminate self-doubt and negative thinking. She needs to focus upon her strengths rather than her limitations. Coach her to select goals and activities that are consistent with her strengths. Too often we lose sight of our strengths because we focus upon our limitations in an effort to be the "perfect person". This puts us in a state of disharmony. Guide her toward recognizing that no one is perfect, and remind her to challenge negative thoughts.

**Investigation:** Suggest that she explore new opportunities. Now is the time for her to be introspective and think about the person she wants to become in this new chapter of her life. It is important that she understands the motives that underlie her actions. Help her to realize that she need not fear what she will find out when she better understands herself. Chances are she will most likely like what she discovers.

**Joy:** Guide her toward learning how to experience joy. Encourage her to become enthusiastic, encouraged and hopeful. Laugh along with her as she laughs out loud. Remember what it was like to be an uninhibited child back when you let yourself go and felt entitled to be happy? Happiness is a relative state not an absolute one. Everything in life does not have to be perfect in order to be happy. Remind her of the positives, and, chances are, they will outweigh the negatives. That is reason enough to feel joy.

**Keepsakes.** Help her search for mementos of her life's journey, benchmarks of her life's progress. It is just as important for her to know where she has been as to know where she is going. This will help her develop a perspective of her personal evolution. Suggest she share with those who are close to her what she has accomplished.

**Love:** Give her enough space to learn to love herself. Be accepting of her, and encourage her to focus on her strengths as opposed to limitations. We often focus on the things that we need to develop (limitations) and lose sight of our strengths. Coach her toward conducting a realistic self-appraisal. Realistic does not mean overly critical. Suggest she give equal balance to strengths and limitations. Do not let her overemphasize the negative.

**Maturity**: Recognize the wisdom and experience that come with maturity. She may need to be reminded during this transition stage that there are many valuable life lessons that have come as a result of living. These lessons are best learned through experience and not through books or others. Maturity is not a euphemism for old.

**Nurturance**: Advise her to look for ways to nurture herself. Suggest that she cultivate "feel good" friendships, volunteer her services to those less fortunate and share the experiences of menopause and other life lessons. Encourage her to give of herself and her experiences.

**Oxygen**: Help her learn to breathe and smell the roses. As she slows down the pace and enjoys the processes as well as the results of her experiences, she will be able to exhale and inhale no matter what stage of life she is in. Her mind will naturally be cleansed when she pays attention to what is good and discards what is not.

**Purpose**: Coach her toward determining what she wants in life. Do the goals that she has set allow her to adapt to changes that may occur? What are the reasons she has set these goals? Guide her toward finding a clear path to enable her to reach her goals. Remind her that it is important to be flexible and to take advantage of the different roads available.

**Questions**: Due to the physiological and psychological reactions that she is experiencing, she may begin to question her competencies. Tell her that such issues as difficulty in maintaining concentration, forgetting something as simple as where she left her keys, and concern about changes in health and general well-being are temporary symptoms of the process and that they disappear with time.

**Resolve**: Now is the time for her to make up her mind to accept who she is, to develop to her potential and discipline herself to work toward reaching her objectives. What her parents, friends, relatives, and others in her life think about her matters much less than what she thinks of herself. In other words, support her as she perseveres toward her goals.

**Strategies:** Guide her as she develops short-range, concrete and challenging objectives to achieve her goals. This is the best strategy to help her remain positive through this transition. The objectives will serve as the pathways for her to achieve her ultimate aspirations. The short-range objectives will serve as the motivators to achieve her ultimate goals; they provide continual reinforcement and a sense of accomplishment along the way. Short-range objectives also provide a history of success.

**Triumphs:** Emphasize her achievements and give her credit where it is due. Too often people lose sight of the accomplishment, no matter how small, and go on to the next objective without giving themselves an opportunity to celebrate achievement. Remind her that she has made it this far and celebrate with her as you both take pride in her successes.

**Understanding:** Help her to make certain that she takes the time to get to know herself. She needs to analyze the impact that she has upon herself and others. Suggest that she pay close attention to the way she feels when she is with others. Ask her if she likes her behavior. Through this analysis she will develop an appreciation of the "why".

**Victories:** By virtue of her reaching this age she has certainly overcome many obstacles. Now is not the time for her to stop setting challenging yet realistic goals. Support her effort to take on meaningful challenges, particularly when there is a strong probability of success. Recommend that she set herself up for rewards that are important to her.

**Wonder:** Coach her to encourage intellectual curiosity. She can appreciate learning for self-satisfaction as opposed to learning just for a test or for a career. Help her to expand her educational horizons by offering support. Suggest she subscribe to a different newspaper, watch The Learning Channel or read a non-fiction book about a topic of interest.

**X—Negativity:** Prompt her to challenge the negatives and self-doubts in her life. Guide her toward working at feeling good. Propose that she make a small change and see how it feels; the next time she can opt for an even greater change. Now is the time for her to take control over something that she can control, her attitude.

**Youthful Outlook**: Age is just a number and there is a distinction between chronological and psychological age. Do not view menopause as the harbinger of the aging process. Psychological age is within our control. If we maintain a youthful positive outlook we can reduce the psychological aging process.

**Zest and Zeal**: Is her glass half-full or half-empty? Work with her at approaching daily activities and long-term goals with a positive and enthusiastic attitude. The power of positive thinking is strong.

# CHAPTER THREE

# LIFE STRATEGY ORIENTATIONS: ASSESSMENTS AND APPROACHES

Women are seen in many different roles—spouse, partner, mother, boss, friend or co-worker. How women are perceived depends on a number of variables: age, race, religion, education, society's expectations and physical characteristics. All of these factors are clearly influential. Less clear, but certainly a significant factor, is that vague concept we typically refer to as personality. Have you ever thought after meeting someone for the first time, that person is not my type, or we do not seem to have too much in common? On the other hand, there are times we meet people and know that we have made a connection.

What happens when the person we have had a relationship with changes? How do we feel when that person behaves very differently from the individual we initially knew? Menopause can result in many personality and behavioral changes that cause the woman we once knew to become a stranger. How can you survive and help her survive the changes that are occurring physiologically and psychologically in her life?

A beginning is to start recognizing the changes that are taking place in your physical and psychological life. Have you noticed that when you visit your physician, he is now requesting a PSA test to measure your prostate health, an electrocardiogram to assess the state of your heart and more extensive blood work to assess conditions that may be age related? What are your feelings and fears regarding the aging process? People at this time begin to recognize their own vulnerability. Understanding your own feelings is the first step in developing empathy for your partner, friend and co-worker.

Key factors that influence our perception of a woman are her temperament and personality characteristics. Therefore, we must recognize some of the essential elements of "personality." An important dynamic of her personality is her **LSO** (Life Strategy Orientation). This refers to the ways that she interacts with the people in her life, gathers information about her world and makes decisions about life events. When you and she are able to understand her **LSO**, you will be better able to help her make her menopausal years "doable." This chapter will help both of you identify her three major **LSOs**[4] (based on Jungian theory).

1. What is her people orientation; is she an Extrovert or an Introvert?

2. How does she gather information about her world and act upon the information; is she a Practical Organized Planner or is she more of a Thoughtful Creative Imaginative?

3. What is her decision-making style; is she an Analytical Issue-Oriented Thinker or an Intuitive People-Oriented Nurturer?

The questionnaires, which follow this section, will identify the various life strategies of the menopausal woman. Responses to the questions which follow this section will help you identify the various **LSOs** of the menopausal woman.

Regardless of a woman's **LSOs**, the physical and emotional changes she experiences during her menopausal years may cause her discomfort and confusion. It is significant to note that although her **LSOs** tend to remain stable over time, there are explicit changes that may occur during menopause. It is important for both of you to recognize that she does not have control over many of these changes. Whether she is your spouse, partner, mother, boss, friend or co-worker, by identifying her life strategies you will both benefit. With a basic understanding of her life strategies before menopause (which you will gain after answering the questionnaire), we will provide you with strategies that will help both of you navigate through menopause. Consider these life strategies as menopause tools that both of you will need to guide you through this transitional time in your lives.

---

[4] One of the most widely used measures of personality preferences, which we call **LSOs**, was originally formulated by Isabel Myers and Katherine Briggs; we have extended their notion of preferences.

## Identification of Life Strategy Orientations (LSOs)

This section includes a questionnaire for you to identify her **LSOs**. You will be introduced to three **LSOs**. These three strategies are key elements in the way we all cope with life and choose the course of action necessary for successful survival. These strategies are:

1. **People Strategy**
2. **Information Gathering and Action Strategy**
3. **Decision Making Strategy**

For each **LSO**, you will be asked to answer questions about behavioral preferences of the menopausal woman in your life. Select the patterns which sound most similar to the choices that you feel she would make. Once you have identified her preference you will be guided to the page where you will find a description of the **LSO**, menopausal reactions for this style, and suggested co-strategies for you to support her as she is coping with these challenges. At the end of the chapter you will find a section labeled Generic Co-strategies. These approaches can be applied to all **LSO**s.

## 1. People Strategy

Instructions: Respond to each question by selecting a yes or no answer.

Is the woman in your life someone that...
- Goes out of her way to meet new people
    Yes(2) No(1)
- Prefers to work alone
    Yes(1) No(2)
- Feels comfortable initiating conversation with strangers
    Yes(2) No(1)
- Waits for others to make the first move in establishing a relationship
    Yes(1) No(2)
- Prefers to surround herself with groups of people
    Yes(2) No(1)
- Is typically quiet and reserved
    Yes(1) No(2)
- Needs to express her thoughts and feelings with others
    Yes(2) No(1)
- Needs time for private reflection of thoughts and feelings
    Yes(1) No(2)

Scoring:  Total the numbers after each of your selections.

If your total score is 14, 15, or 16, her People Orientation is Extrovert. Her section starts on the following page.

If your total score is 8, 9, or 10, her People Orientation is Introvert. This section begins on page 29.

If your total score is 11, 12, or 13, her People Orientation is a blend of both Introvert and Extrovert.

For the blend, read the **LSO**s of Extrovert and Introvert selecting the characteristics that best describe her.

# Extroverts are:

- Social
- Expressive
- Interactive
- Outward
- Prone to action before thinking

The Extrovert gets her energy from the outer world and tends to feel drained when she spends too much time by herself. We know that Extroverts become charged up by contact with people. Because she usually experiences a surge of energy when she is with others, she is quick to approach others (even strangers) and feels comfortable initiating a conversation. Such interaction charges the Extrovert's batteries and makes her feel alive. This does not necessarily indicate that individuals, who score high on the Extrovert scale, are more outgoing and lively than others. It simply suggests that everything they do relates to the outside world. Generally, the Extrovert is gregarious and enjoys meeting a lot of different people, and she feels energized by the experience. An Extrovert wants to stay at a party until the bitter end and then go on to another. Extroverts tend to be expressive, and individuals who are expressive appear more comfortable around groups of people than they are when alone. Not only do Extroverts talk more than Introverts, but they also are more comfortable communicating their feelings, emotional states, and experiences to others. Extroverts tend to say what is on their minds, almost as though they were thinking out loud. The expressive individual is quick to speak and slow to listen because she is so eager to tell others what she is thinking. So, if the woman in your life:

- Talks more than she listens
- Communicates with a great deal of enthusiasm
- Is distracted easily
- Meets people readily and enjoys participating in many different activities
- Tends to blurt things out without thinking

- Is always on the go
- Likes working in groups or teams
- Enjoys being the center of attention

she is high on the Extrovert scale and receives her flow of energy from external sources.

## The Extrovert's Reactions to Menopause

Prior to menopause, the Extrovert had always been the "life of the party". She generally did not want to spend time alone. When you and she returned home from work at the end of the day her energy level appeared to be greater than at the beginning of the day. She could not wait to talk to you about the events and people she had encountered. She talked about all of her co-workers as though they were her close friends. She complained about being bored when she was inactive for too long and looked for opportunities where she was the center of attention. She was "turned on" by meeting new people and exploring new places and loved discussing the events in her life.

Lately however, the woman whom you have always believed to have a thick skin cries at the drop of a hat, chooses to isolate herself from others and appears sensitive to more issues than she has in the past. She feels threatened by new situations, people and even her friends. While she used to be your sounding board at the end of your long day, she no longer gives you the time she once did. With the change her body is undergoing, caused by menopause, she does not have the energy that she previously had. She is not able to "charge her batteries" using the same methods as she did before menopause.

Before menopause, when she was anxious or depressed, she was able to manage these feelings by connecting herself with other people or busying herself with various activities. Menopause has depleted so much of her energy that she often finds interaction with people and her daily activities draining her batteries rather than recharging them. Fatigue sets in easily, and whereas she used to ignore being tired and keep on going, she no longer can.

She has a wide network of friends upon whom she has always relied to share her personal information. However, she may now be experiencing new insecurities resulting in suspicion and jealousy that may preclude her from seeking out her old friends or making new ones. These new insecurities, experienced by many menopausal women, coupled with constant fatigue from lack of sleep due to hot flashes, adds up to emotional and physical distress. When she looks in the mirror she may not see the woman she remembers. Instead she focuses on the subtle changes, new wrinkles, gray hairs and sunspots. Her clothes fit differently, and she finds it difficult to remember the last time she received a compliment about her looks or a second glance from a male stranger on the street. Being the center of attention and laughing at her own faults has always been her trademark. Now that she is going through "the change," you notice that she laughs less and spends more time in front of the mirror noticing her body than ever before. She has a hard time laughing at her dry skin and thinning hair. The exercises that were her panacea for a flabby stomach may no longer work. Her stomach may sag more, even though she is exercising more. She may surprise you by deciding not to attend her annual holiday party because she is feeling uncomfortable about how she looks. Some menopausal women even avoid the grocery store, fearful that they might run into someone they know, when in the past this was a social event. Your thick-skinned Extrovert, the woman in your life who has always been able to take a joke, is having a difficult time getting through the day.

So how does a woman who thrives on being in the company of others survive with these new feelings of fear, suspicion, jealously and body changes?

## She Does, He Does…Co-strategies for the Extrovert

- Encourage her to talk about what she is feeling. The Extrovert, by simply expressing her feelings, finds the outlet she needs to use some of her energy. In addition to helping her vent some of her stored up energies you are also able to show her your concern by listening to what she has to say. Ask her direct questions about issues that are of concern. When you respond to her answers, if she happens to make statements like "you just don't understand," ask her to help you understand. Listen carefully to what she is telling you. Try not to make statements like, "That is ridiculous," or "Listen to how crazy that sounds." Allow her to verbalize her concerns without making light of them.

- Maintain good eye contact with her as she speaks to you and make sure the television and radio are off so there are no distractions. To make certain you have heard what she is feeling and you understand her primary concerns, rephrase what she has told you and ask her if you understood her correctly. By rephrasing you are showing her you have listened and you are giving her the opportunity to clarify any misconceptions. Be patient by allowing her to finish her thoughts and show her your support with a calming voice.

- The Extrovert needs to express herself. Do not shut her out, even if what she is saying seems unreasonable to you. If it seems to you that she is not enjoying herself as much as she used to with some of her friends, ask her which of her friends she feels most comfortable with and let her know it is all right with you to be with whomever she wants.

- You know the old cliché "keep the lines of communication open"? Now, during this transitional period, it is more important than ever before to follow this adage. In the past you and she may have enjoyed lively discussions about the events of the day, but now she needs to talk about her new feelings. Give her the time to express herself. But also remember to ask her for time for you to express your feelings. Communication involves a sender and a receiver of a message. Be certain to switch roles so you have your chance at being the sender.

## Introverts are:

- Private
- Quiet
- Contemplative
- Inward
- Prone to thinking before acting

The Introvert gets her energy from within and quickly loses her energy when having to deal with a lot of people. In order for the Introvert to charge up her battery, she needs quiet and solitude. This does not mean that Introverts are shy, quiet and withdrawn, it means that they are generally introspective, they go "inside themselves" to think things through before they react to a situation or respond to a question. Introverts need a lot of time to themselves. Rather than approach a stranger, the Introvert will wait until someone approaches her. An Introvert is generally an individual of "few words". She is quite reserved and tends to be comfortable when alone, inclined to pursue solitary activities. This does not mean that she does not enjoy the company of others—quite the contrary. She does enjoy socializing, but at large social gatherings or meetings she tends to find a quiet corner where she can converse with just one or possibly two others. So, if the woman in your life:

- Avoids crowds and looks for quiet
- Listens more than talks
- Is not easily distracted
- Is cautious in meeting people and participates in one activity at a time
- Thinks carefully before speaking
- Needs alone time to reflect
- Prefers to work alone or socialize in small groups
- Is content being on the sidelines

she is high on the Introvert scale and derives her energy from within.

## The Introvert's Reactions to Menopause

The Introvert has always enjoyed her private time. When the phone rings and she is at home alone, chances are she will let the answering machine record the message. If you are at home, she will wait for you to answer the phone. Prior to menopause her mode of communication had characteristically been through serious conversations involving just the two of you. She developed a few very close friendships, and she was extremely devoted to those friends. As a matter of fact, she was such a devoted person that her friends were generally lifetime friends. You may be aware that she was the type of individual who always took her time before responding to a question or making a decision. Most of the time she rehearsed things before saying them and often responded to a question with, "I'll have to think about that". If there was a crowd, she did not engage in conversation, but retreated to a quiet corner of the room in order to find one or two others to share in a discussion. She did not need the approval of others because she was able to seek approval from herself.

Prior to menopause, she was always able to work things out on her own without sharing her worries or concerns with others. But when her heart starts racing and fluctuating hormone levels cause her to have bouts of anxious feelings, she has a difficult time dealing with anxiety. This feeling may cause her concern. Her caution in sharing with others may force her to retreat further into herself to work out her anxiety and she may appear even more withdrawn, perhaps antisocial.

The fatigue she may feel due to lack of sleep caused by fluctuating hormone levels sets her back even further, because she may have a difficult time concentrating. She has always taken pride in the knowledge that she is aware of what is going on inside her mind and body. Now that has all changed. She is frightened by what is happening, but keeps her fears locked up inside.

The woman in your life who is an Introvert has always had a few intimate friends, those to whom she is extremely devoted. She knows that she can rely on these friends and shares her thoughts and feelings with them (Most of them are Introverts as well). However, some of the symptoms of menopause have caused a change in how she views these friendships, and this is especially disturbing to the Introvert, who is an extremely faithful friend. The bouts of suspicion and jealousy she is feeling due to lack of sleep and hormonal changes are challenging her feelings of devotion. She is not sure whether or not she can trust her dear friends, and this leaves her totally alone. In addition, she may experience short-term memory loss due to hormonal fluctuations. This causes a great deal of distress for the woman who prides herself on working alone and relying almost entirely on herself for decisions. The Introvert who is typically shy and reserved retreats even further away from those who are closest to her.

She is concerned about the change her body is undergoing as she reaches menopause. The new wrinkle that appears overnight, the gray and thinning hair that her hairdresser points out and the thickening around her waist affect the way she feels about herself. Because the Introvert tends to work her problems out inwardly, she may never let you know how she truly feels about these menopausal changes. The frequent and quick mood changes she is experiencing, probably for the first time in her life, are worrisome for the Introverted menopausal woman, and the solitude she has always needed to get through the day is not helping her recharge her batteries. She finds herself in total isolation. Her previous coping mechanisms, seeking privacy and peace, are not providing her with the positive results she expects.

## She Does, He Does…Co-strategies for the Introvert

- Value her privacy. Do not invade the space she needs although you may want to be with her. She needs to conserve her personal energy, so help her by providing an opportunity for her to be home alone. Let her know you respect her needs and schedule one night a week out of the house to give her the privacy she needs. Take your son or daughter to dinner and a movie or go to the library and catch up on newspapers or magazines you have not read. Make arrangements to go to a sporting event with a work colleague. Whatever you decide to do, make certain to let her know you have regard for her need for privacy.

- Encourage her to take the private time she needs for herself to recharge her batteries. This may require finding personal space at home for her to "be with herself" without distractions: away from the television, interruptions of the telephone and other demands of the household.

- While respecting her need for privacy and giving her space, also let her know you think it would be enjoyable to socialize with another couple. If you feel as though she does not want to socialize with another couple, just the two of you go out for dinner and to the movies. However, it is useful to encourage her to socialize with others because this serves as an opportunity to shift her attention from herself and direct it to others. Offer specific plans and ask for her input. Remember to follow the pace for activities that works for her and avoid any form of criticism, regardless of whether you believe her pace is too slow.

Understanding the Introvert's need to be introspective and private, suggest she record her memoirs in a personal journal. This chronicle provides her the opportunity to record her daily thoughts and feelings and process what is happening to her due to menopause.

## 2. Information Gathering and Action Strategy

Instructions: Respond to each question by selecting a yes or no answer.

Is the woman in your life is someone that…

- Prefers days that are unplanned and casual
  Yes(2)   No(1)
- Reads and follows instructions carefully
  Yes(1)   No(2)
- Likes her day to have a variety of tasks and activities
  Yes(2)   No(1)
- Prefers to give detailed instructions to accomplish a task
  Yes(1)   No(2)
- Enjoys change and new situations
  Yes(2)   No(1)
- Is orderly and systematic
  Yes(1)   No(2)
- Begins many projects and may not finish them
  Yes(2)   No(1)
- Is comfortable with her routine
  Yes(1)   No(2)

Scoring:   Total the numbers after your selections.

If your total score is 8, 9 or 10, her information gathering and action orientation is Practical Organized Planner. Her section starts on the following page.

If your total score is 14, 15 or 16, her information gathering and action orientation is Thoughtful Creative Imaginative. You will find this section on page 38.

If your total score is 11, 12 or 13, her information gathering and action orientation is a blend of Practical Organized Planner and Thoughtful Creative Imaginative. Read the LSO of Practical Organized Planner and Thoughtful Creative Imaginative selecting the characteristics that best describe her.

## The Practical Organized Planner is:

- Well organized
- Detail oriented
- Realistic
- Efficient
- Practical

The Practical Organized Planner is an individual who prefers to live in a well-organized and orderly world. She tends to see what is rather than what might be; her information is gained primarily by her five senses.

She looks at objects to see them, listens to sounds to hear them, touches surfaces to feel them, sniffs odors to smell them, and mouths substances to taste them. Her style in approaching life is to establish goals, defining them with clarity and specificity. She proceeds to work with her energy, focus and concentration to reach her goals. She cares about facts and details rather than possibilities. She tends to pay closer attention to what is going on outside of herself, that is, being mindful of the external environment rather than listening to the inner self. As a pragmatic planner, she tends to communicate in a direct way. She strives for clarification and detail to see matters clearly and is most inclined to feel comfortable attending to the particulars of everyday living and concrete things such as food, shelter and clothing. Friends and family describe her as "solid, trustworthy and dependable". Although she is down to earth and sees what is "now," she pays close attention to details and does not miss what is happening. So, if the woman in your life:

- Prefers living with a structure that has a beginning, middle and end
- Tends to be specific and literal and gives detailed descriptions
- Behaves practically
- Is methodical
- Likes predictability
- Sets goals and works methodically towards them
- Likes to see things in clear and well defined terms
- Values realism and common sense

she is high on the Practical Organized Planner scale, gathers information about her world through her five senses and prefers to live in a structured and organized way.

## The Practical Organized Planner's Reaction to Menopause

The Practical Organized Planner is known by her friends and relatives as the woman who can do anything. The bouts of emotion that may accompany menopause are very frustrating and confusing, as they may distract and disrupt her from her very scheduled life. Because she sees what is directly in front of her and is incredibly attuned to details, she feels that these roller coaster highs and lows prevent her from her focused and organized lifestyle. Her previous, indefatigable manner is greatly compromised by these symptoms, and as a result, she may feel irritable, an emotion she directs at anybody and anything in her path. She craves information, trusts facts and has a keen memory. The physical symptoms, including hot flashes, headaches and menstrual irregularities cause her to detour from her personal agenda and well-defined goals and objectives, which may intensify her frustration, creating irritability and a critical nature.

This is a woman who has always prided herself on the ability to be organized, punctual and focused. One of the traits that is so appealing to those who associate with her is the practical way in which she deals with situations. However, her recent memory blips, caused by menopause, are some of the most distressing changes that the Practical Organized Planner experiences. She may spend an incredibly frustrating 20 seconds in between the stove and the refrigerator, while preparing dinner, knowing she needs an additional onion for the dish she is preparing as she heads to the refrigerator, but forgetting it is the onion she needs by the time she gets there. Menopause can also challenge her long-term memory. She who relies on her past experiences to assist in making present day decisions feels a great deal of frustration when she cannot depend on her recall. Imagine how exasperating it can feel to lose your method of gathering information about your world.

The Practical Organized Planner tends to think sequentially, from A to B to C, using inductive reasoning (going from the specific to the general). While in the throes of menopause, it may be extremely difficult for her to focus on one thing at a time, and she may not feel confident about her thinking skills. She may face the continual challenge of wondering if she will forget a word in the middle of a sentence or lose track of time.

As the Practical Organized Planner has been a woman who has demanded much of herself, she may have great difficulty accepting the changes that are happening to her body and mind. She may initially find ways to resist these changes or deny they are occurring, blaming them on outside causes. These are the times that will be most trying for friends, family members and work colleagues who are a part of her life.

## She Does, He Does......Co-strategies for the Practical Organized Planner

- Now it is time to reevaluate. Maybe this is when you need to discuss changes in your household that might lighten her responsibility load. When you begin to see signs of her frustration in her ability to accomplish tasks, the results of which may be displaced on you, rather than reacting in kind, attempt to be patient and understanding. Recognize that she needs your assistance and do not respond defensively. Suggest making a to-do list together. Maybe it is time to consider reassignment of household tasks. Perhaps it is time to hire household or garden maintenance services.

- Remember that she needs facts and data that are presented with explicit detail in order to organize her thoughts. Consider Sunday brunch as a time to discuss the calendar for the upcoming week: her activities, your activities and shared activities. This time spent providing her with the weekly overview may provide her with all the information she needs for an organized and well-planned week.

- Be her partner by making it easier for her to manage this transition phase. Research information sources relating to menopause, e.g. the internet, the library, bookstores. Increase your knowledge and understanding of menopausal issues so that you become a credible sounding board and resource for her.

- Work with her to establish realistic goal expectations by teaching her to say "no," and assure her that it is often appropriate to say "no." Reassure her that saying "no" is really ok and that she has to understand what her new boundaries are in terms of time and energy.

## The Thoughtful Creative Imaginative is:

- Spontaneous
- Innovative
- Flexible
- Change-oriented
- Open to new possibilities

The Thoughtful Creative Imaginative tends to rely on her instincts to take in information about her world. She listens to her inner voice and pays close attention to what is going on inside herself. She is happiest when her life is flexible and open to new possibilities. She enjoys her day the most when it is full of variety, spontaneity and adventure. She is described by individuals who live or work with her as the "Queen of Multi-tasking." Her activities tend to be geared toward those that require creativity, and she generally looks at the bigger picture, rather than focusing in on the details of everyday life. This is the woman who enjoys keeping all of her options open. As a result, it is not at all unusual for her to change her goals as she receives new information. She begins each new endeavor with unbridled energy and enthusiasm, but as the activity begins to not be new, she may become distracted by something else and abandon the project midstream. Endings and completions are not as central to her life as the start and new beginnings of projects. So if the woman in your life:

- Focuses on possibilities
- Likes to begin new projects, but procrastinates finishing
- Changes goals in the middle of a project
- Has a workspace that may appear somewhat disorganized
- Is limitless with ways to solve problems
- Values imagination and innovation
- Works from an abstract sense of values
- Enjoys creative activity

she is high on the Thoughtful Creative Imaginative scale and prefers a lifestyle of spontaneity and flexibility while gathering information about her world through intuition.

# The Thoughtful Creative Imaginative's Reaction to Menopause

The Thoughtful Creative Imaginative considers herself the "big picture" person, looking for the creative and flexible approach to life situations. She enjoys managing a full range of activities in a very casual, flexible and spontaneous manner. The many changes that accompany menopause, including rapidly fluctuating emotions, fatigue and mental lapses, make it more difficult for her to manage her life effectively. Prior to menopause she was able to keep her schedule and daily tasks well controlled with her casual style. However, now she is experiencing frustration and confusion. She finds she has planned two activities at the same time, or she shows up for a doctor's appointment at the right time but on the wrong day, or she bounces a couple of checks because she forgot to record previous expenditures. In the past she found that making lists was an unnecessary task. Her mental shopping list was readily available and she accomplished what was necessary. That is no longer true.

Time is relative to the Thoughtful Creative Imaginative. She may have difficulty keeping on task or following explicit directions. She can spend a lot of time daydreaming in her fantasy world and looking toward future possibilities. She may be great at interpreting facts or gathering insights and has little interest in details. She most likely tends to look for underlying patterns by using her sixth sense, intuition.

Menopausal symptoms create a great challenge for the philosophical, conceptual idealist. The woman who is used to getting information about her world through creative approaches may be thwarted due to menopausal symptoms such as migraines, hot flashes, and anxiety. Worries about the physical manifestations of menopause are overwhelming to the woman who has always trusted her intuitive powers. Her body is telling her to pay attention, but her mind says let us first consider what is happening in an abstract manner. Perhaps for the first time in her life she must deal with what is "now".

Prior to menopause she had many theories about life situations and enjoyed figuring things out just for the sake of figuring them out. She liked to adjust and dabble with her theories, looking at them very philosophically and constantly asking herself what things meant on a larger scale. However, the physical and emotional changes brought on by shifting hormone levels are wreaking havoc on her worldview. She cannot concentrate on any thought long enough to develop a theory. When she is able to develop a creative approach, she may have a memory blip and lose her train of thought. Deductive reasoning (going from the general to the specific), the method she has always used to gather information about her world, has come to a screeching halt.

Although time has always been relative to the philosophical, conceptual big picture, the fatigue factor, caused by fluctuating hormone levels, precludes her from moving faster than a snail's pace. She may enthusiastically accept a dinner invitation, only to be unable to get herself motivated to get to the dinner. When she finally does arrive, the party is just about over, and she feels bad about having disappointed the host. However, she finds herself in the same situation with the next invitation.

Before experiencing menopausal symptoms, she always had faith in her hunches and drew on the unknown, the indirect and the not-yet-experienced. Now she is finding that her quick mood changes and frequent fatigue are getting in the way of her intuitions, hindering the only way she is accustomed to gathering information about her world.

## She Does, He Does...Co-strategies for the Thoughtful Creative Imaginative

- Control your frustration. The fact is that tasks which she managed in a casual way before are now being addressed in an even less organized manner, or even neglected. She may be experiencing a sense of alarm at not being able to remember a simple telephone message. Display as much patience as possible by letting her know you will work with her. Take it upon yourself to create an environment to help her with the simple chores. Purchase pads and pencils and put them next to each telephone in the house. Leave her notes on the pad so she gets used to the idea of messages. These tools will allow her to feel the sense of organization she needs through this transitional time.

- Because she is a "big picture" person try not to get bogged down with the details of a situation. Help her through this period by organizing all the "little" things in your lives. Sit with her and make out a shopping list and remind her to take it to the supermarket. Praise her when she completes the chore you have spoken about. Do not discourage her from her philosophical orientation. Recognize that by using these strategies she will get the reassurance and the support that will outlast this transitional period of menopause.

- Enable her to see the "bigger picture" of menopause. Shift the focus of this evolutionary change from "what was" to "what will be," reminding her that the best is yet to come. Support her new way of processing her changing world, and encourage her to try out some new roles. Has there been a career dream that she put on hold while she was raising a family or because she sensed financial restrictions? This is your chance to encourage her pursuits in new personal interests. With your support and encouragement her new focus will be a celebration of her independent, unique and individual style.

- Listen to her and show interest in her ideas. Strive to build up her level of confidence by responding positively to her views. Paraphrase or summarize by restating the content of her message and be sensitive to the level of emotion that may be reflected. This will affirm her new way of processing her changing world and give her the opportunity of using you as a sounding board.

- It is important to recognize that she is not looking to you for answers but rather to be a part of the process of developing strategies to help her navigate through the transitional stage of menopause. Take her concerns seriously. She lives her life using deductive reasoning (going from the general to the specific) and needs to reason from this perspective. She knows what she feels but not why. Work with her to help her figure out the why. Use analogies and metaphors when talking with her. Compare and contrast what she is feeling now versus what she felt before she experienced the symptoms of menopause.

## 3. Decision Making Strategy

Is the woman in your life someone that...

- Bases decisions more on facts that feelings
      Yes(1)  No(2)
- Bases decisions more on feelings than facts
      Yes(2)  No(1)
- Is critical of people and situations
      Yes(1)  No(2)
- Is concerned about maintaining peace and harmony
      Yes(2)  No(1)
- Appears blunt and tactless on occasion
      Yes(1)  No(2)
- Thrives on praise from others
      Yes(2)  No(1)
- Enjoys problem solving activities
      Yes(1)  No(2)
- Likes doing things to please others
      Yes(2)  No(1)

Scoring:   Total the numbers after your selections.

If your total score is 8, 9 or 10, her decision-making orientation is Analytical Issue-Oriented Thinker. Her section begins on the following page.

If your total score is 14, 15 or 16, her decision-making orientation is Intuitive People-Oriented Nurturer. This section begins on page 47.

If your total score is 11, 12 or 13, her decision-making orientation is a blend of both Analytical Issue-Oriented Thinker and Intuitive People-Oriented Nurturer. For the blend, read the **LSO**s of Analytical Issue-Oriented Thinker and Intuitive People-Oriented Nurturer selecting the characteristics that best describe her.

For the blend, read the **LSO**s of Analytical Issue-Oriented Thinker and Intuitive People-Oriented Nurturer, selecting the characteristics that are descriptive of the woman in your life.

## The Analytical Issue-Oriented Thinker is:

- Logical
- Methodical
- Objective
- Rational
- Emotionally Controlled

The Analytical Issue-Oriented Thinker approaches decisions in her life in a very logical, methodical manner. She likes to take a step back from the situation and analyze it thoroughly before making her factually based decision. Her decisions are reached by carefully considering all evidence available, and she will arrive at an objective conclusion, even when the results of her decision bring unpleasant or negative consequences. Her personal decision-making standard is to apply logic, justice and fairness consistently—to each and every situation and each and every individual. As she values the analytical process and the truth, she at times can be seen by her friends, family members and work colleagues as tactless, heartless, insensitive and uncaring. A friend or loved one may even be heard to say, "She is honest to a fault, always truthful but not very tactful or diplomatic."

She is also a keen observer with a shrewd, analytical eye. People who know her will conclude that she never misses anything, and you surely cannot get anything past her. Along with her acute observational ability comes her attention to flaws or imperfections. She does not hesitate to pass this feedback on to those around her, and this tends to make others perceive her as critical. For her, this "constructive criticism" (as she characterizes it) is motivated by her desire for achievement, accomplishment and excellence, which are central to her sense of self.

So, if the woman in your life:
- Prides herself on being an objective, logical thinker
- Makes decisions impersonally
- Bases decisions primarily on facts

- Weighs the evidence carefully and thoroughly before making a decision
- Can be described as straightforward and critical
- Values directness and honesty
- Is motivated by a need for achievement and accomplishment
- Is acutely aware of her environment

She is high on the Analytical Issue-Oriented thinking scale and interacts with the world and takes in information in a very methodical and analytical way.

## The Analytical Issue-Oriented Thinker's Reactions to Menopause

The Thinker is the woman who has always prided herself on approaching life's challenges and decisions from a very logical, analytical and methodical style. At the first signs of menopausal symptoms there may be a tendency to ignore and deny both physical and psychological changes. She may attempt to explain these changes in terms of temporary life situations, e.g. stress at work, or a new virus strain. As the thinker tends to be a perfectionist, both self-critical and critical of others, these characteristics may become even more dramatic. She may become increasingly impatient and more demanding of herself and others, and this may spill over to friends, family and colleagues. As these characteristics become even more pronounced, she may be perceived as cold and detached by others. As someone who has previously been seen as not needing others, she may experience difficulty in getting the support from others that she requires at this time. A conflict may emerge between her new needs for support from others and the prevailing view that she is pushing others away. This conflict may also manifest itself internally, as she becomes aware of these new feelings. She has always felt very confident and self-assured and these new feelings may cause her to wrestle with self-doubt. As she becomes accepting of the fact that she is menopausal, her next strategy may be to search far and wide for the latest information and appropriate treatments of menopausal symptoms. As she is typically impatient, she may experience increased frustration due to the paucity of available information and available treatments.

## She Does, He Does...Co-strategies for the Analytical Issue-Oriented Thinker

- Initiate conversations about her feelings and the possible reasons for them. You may have observed changes in the way she expresses herself. Since feelings are often unexplored territory for her, she may experience a sense of confusion and an inability to articulate what she is feeling. It will require gentle invitations for the expression of these feelings. Concern and constancy will provide her a safe environment to connect with the feelings she has had difficulty articulating. This process will help her develop insight into the underlying reasons for these behavioral changes.

- Curb the impulse to tell her to lighten up, to stop taking life so seriously and to quit hassling you. Doing so would only exacerbate the situation and escalate her perfectionism and critical nature to an even higher level. Try the strategy of counting to 10 and giving yourself a chance to focus before responding to her.

- Encourage her to reach out to friends and relatives during this transitional time. Because she does not readily ask for help, on a psychological or physical level, let her know that it is all right to do so. Suggest discussion groups that typically talk about women's issues. Subscribe to magazines for her that publish articles relating to menopausal issues—the difficulty women have dealing with menopausal symptoms and the effect they have on their lives.

- Assure her that she has not lost her skills, that any lapses are merely temporary in nature and that her self-confidence will return when she has completed this transitional period. Discuss with her issues relating to events that interested her in the past, perhaps find a thought-provoking article in a magazine or newspaper that you feel might interest her and spend time talking about it.

## The Intuitive People-Oriented Nurturer is:

- Empathic
- Supportive
- Cooperative
- Emotional
- Loyal

The Intuitive People-Oriented Nurturer approaches life with a desire to create harmony in all aspects of her life. Whenever she is in a situation that requires a decision or an action to be taken, she always considers first how others will feel and will be affected by the decision or action. After doing so, her decision will be based on what she feels is right and what she cares about the most. As a result, at times her concern and feelings about the individuals affected by the decision may outweigh logic and facts. Her strengths are clearly shown in her ability to be empathic and compassionate to all around her. She very much values these attributes, and they tend to be central to her sense of self. Sometimes others experience this woman's decision-making style as irrational. However, it is a rational approach in which the feeling component takes priority over the factual and logical components. This woman may be described as "someone who wears her heart on her sleeve," as she is greatly affected by the emotional content of all situations. She would never be identified as a "poker face", since by just looking at her, you will know what she is feeling at any time. As a result of her preference for the feeling aspects of a situation, sometimes her friends, family and work colleagues may perceive her as a bit overemotional. She is extremely sensitive to the comments and criticisms of those around her. She does gain much personal pleasure from pleasing others and expresses her appreciation of your efforts and contributions to any situation. Tact is very much a virtue for her, and she will work very hard to communicate difficult information in the most diplomatic manner. She may even avoid handling difficult situations in order not to hurt or offend anyone else. Her most valued accomplishments are those that gain the appreciation of friends, family and work colleagues. So, if the woman in your life:

- Establishes warm and friendly relationships with others
- Is available to listen to others' complaints
- Supports others' feelings
- Is a ready friend and advocate for others
- Receives satisfaction from pleasing others and receiving approval
- Enjoys harmonious environments free of conflict
- Tends to idealize others
- Enjoys helping others grow and develop

She is high on the intuitive people-oriented nurturing scale and prefers to make decisions based on what she cares about, rather than on analyzing and weighing the evidence.

## The Intuitive People-Oriented Nurturer's Reactions to Menopause

The Nurturer has spent most of her life energy and time attending to the needs and feelings of others. Since she has been so focused on others, there is a distinct possibility for self-neglect, which may lead to a significant period of crankiness and irritability during this stage. Another result of spending so much time focusing on the needs of others in her life may be that she is now experiencing "empty nest syndrome"—a period of sadness as her children separate from home and establish their own independence. She may also be experiencing burnout from her continued role as a caretaker at home, in her career and in her community service activities. She may feel exhausted about attempting to find ways to care for her aging parents, or she may be struggling with the loss of her parents. As the Nurturer is already a woman for whom feelings have been a very important part of her life, the hormonal changes accompanying menopause may intensify her feelings and heighten her sensitivity to comments and behaviors of colleagues, friends, and loved ones.

## She Does, He Does…Co-strategies for the Intuitive People-Oriented Nurturer

- Encourage her to shift her attention from caring about others to caring about herself and her personal needs. Maybe it is a good time to suggest some new activities for her to pursue, which will encourage her individual development. This may be the first time she has thought of herself at center stage. Perhaps you can suggest courses at a university, yoga, photography, cooking, tennis or golf, working with a personal trainer or regular visits to a spa.

- Take this opportunity to put your relationship at the center of her attention. Suggest evening walks together, dance lessons, a quiet weekend away. Maybe it is even a time to plan a second honeymoon. All strategies are designed to help her feel positive about herself and to reenergize your relationship. Can you surprise her with a romantic dinner at home or at her favorite restaurant? These novel ways can improve the quality of her life and your marriage during this evolutional life stage.

- Guide and support her in defining limits and boundaries in terms of meeting others' needs and expectations. The needs of aging parents may cause her to feel increased responsibility. The children may expect her to be the perennial babysitter, or her boss may see her as the individual who can never say "no" to the extra assignment. Suggest that she maintain a daily planner with allocated time for herself and your relationship. Make certain that this time is viewed as sacrosanct and cannot be usurped by the needs of others. Remind her that it is appropriate to put you and your relationship as a top priority.

- Provide a calming, reassuring, focused communication style, which focuses more on issues than feelings. Nurturers tend to process information and resolve problems as they speak. At times, she may appear to be overly emotional, and it may be necessary to ground her in the issues and facts she needs to attend to. This may give her a greater sense of control and accomplishable tasks.

## General Co-Strategies

- Be an active partner through this transitional stage of your lives. Although you cannot experience menopause and its symptoms with her you can be there to share the process with her. Attempt to be empathetic and, as she expresses the various physical and psychological changes she is experiencing, try to put yourself in her shoes. Indeed, how would it feel to endure hot flashes, sleepless nights and memory blips? Be a true partner, and spend some time reading about menopause so you can be aware of what is happening to her. Tell her you want to accompany her to a doctor's appointment, if she so chooses, because you care about her and you want to learn about menopause so you can understand from a male perspective what she is going through.

- Work hard at helping her to understand that you plan to stand by her through this period of transition. If you have not spent a lot of leisure time together in the past, and you do not plan on changing, compensate by finding the words that will communicate how much you care.

- Go to the bookstore together and pull books about menopause off the shelf. Look for books that talk about menopause in a humorous way so you and your partner can unwind with a good laugh. You will find that there are books filled with cartoons and humorous stories about menopause. Sit at one of the tables in the bookstore and look through the books together. Encourage her to purchase one or two of the books that appear appropriate for your lives. If she is hesitant to sit at the bookstore with you, go to the bookstore on your way home from work, purchase a couple of books about menopause and bring them home to her. Secure a time when both of you can go through the books together. Discuss what you have read and ask her if she is experiencing many or some of the symptoms the books talk about.

- Try to increase the amount of time you spend together. Share quiet dinners, movies, walking around the block after dinner, golfing, bowling, whatever your choice. During your time alone reassure her how important she is in your life and express how much you care about her.

- What you have done in the past to help her feel attractive may not work during this transitional stage. Be sensitive to what she articulates about the changes and try to minimize what she views as negative, e.g. weight gain, new wrinkles, age spots. Encourage her to do those things that make her feel good and sexy e.g. a manicure or a pedicure. Purchasing a new outfit and wearing it to dinner or to an evening at a friend's house may do the trick (as long as you compliment her new clothes).

- Encourage communication that makes each of you aware of what you find attractive in each other in order to maintain the "spice" in your relationship. The day that she is wearing the dress that you have always liked go out of your way to compliment her. If she is wearing a particular perfume that you like, surprise her with a bottle as a gift. It will serve as a clear message for her to wear it again!

- Request that she communicate with you regarding the various choices you make concerning your clothing and personal grooming. If she finds something particularly attractive, make it a point to wear it more frequently and inform her that it is because she likes it.

- She may not want to make love because she feels uncomfortable with her body and she no longer feels attractive. Perhaps she is embarrassed with her "changed" menopausal look and does not want you to see her unclothed. Maybe intercourse is painful due to menopausal symptoms. It is up to you to let her know you still find her attractive and want to be with her. If intercourse is painful, she needs to know that there are creams and lotions she can use to help alleviate what may be causing the discomfort. Discuss alternate ways to make love and satisfy each other.

- Encourage her to remain as active as she had been prior to menopause. To let her know you understand that her energy level may be compromised, suggest she modify certain activities rather than eliminate them from her routine.

- Take on the role of social event coordinator, if necessary. Pull out the newspaper and suggest a movie. Ask her if she would like you to call friends to find out if they are free and would like to join the two of you for movies and a bite to eat afterwards. Treat it like a date night, and do not forget to compliment her outfit, hair or shoes.

- Spend time just holding her. The fact that she may have a difficult time verbalizing what she is feeling does not mean she does not want you near. Do not force her to talk to you when you sense she needs to be quiet. This has nothing to do with you; it is all about the "change" that she is experiencing. She still wants and needs to be loved and cared for by you.

- She may feel unattractive because her clothes fit differently or her hair is thinner and it does not "work" for her the way it did before menopause. Show her how you still find her attractive. Buy a rose on the way home from work and surprise her with it when you arrive home. Tell her it is "simply because."

- If she tells you she feels fat let her know you do not think she is. If you believe she has gained some weight offer some suggestions. Tell her that a certain degree of weight gain can be expected during the menopausal process, however if she is still concerned, the following strategies might be appropriate to consider. Ask her if she would like to start an exercise routine with you. Consider low caloric ways of preparing food. You might suggest membership in a gym or purchasing exercise equipment for your home. Consider taking a walk together after dinner a few times a week. Perhaps Weight Watchers or another diet management program would be an effective alternative.

- This is the time to anticipate that she may be overly sensitive and she may distort or misinterpret some of the things you say. You can cope with distortion in communication by utilizing the concept of redundancy (over communicating by including in the message additional elements which are not strictly essential for its understanding). With the use of phrases like, "in other words" or "for instance," you may reduce miscommunication. It does not mean saying the same thing twice, but paraphrasing the message because the receiver may be in a stressful or anxious state. It may be useful to restate the message and to provide relevant examples in order to facilitate understanding.

# CHAPTER FOUR

# WHERE ARE WE NOW AND WHERE DO WE GO FROM HERE?

You have the necessary "tools" to make the menopausal process better. Now we are going to present you with some common situations/scenarios that you may be confronted with during this process. Along with these scenarios is a choice of strategies for you to choose from that can make these situations better or make them worse. We have confidence that you will be able to choose the techniques that will make the situation better; after all you now know how to "step into her shoes."

## Scenario 1

Your partner is experiencing a hot flash while you are together at a social gathering. You notice that she is perspiring and her makeup is running down her face; her hair has droplets of water; she is drenched with sweat. It is obvious to you that she is feeling extremely uncomfortable.

| How to Make the Situation Better | How to Make the Situation Worse |
|---|---|
| • Suggest that you go to a quiet corner | • Tell her that you think it is best if you both leave because she is drawing attention to herself |
| • Offer to get her a cold drink | • Ignore the situation |

- Tell her that you understand if she wants to leave

- Tell her to go to the restroom and take care of herself

## Scenario 2

Your partner begins to cry for no apparent reason.

### How to Make the Situation Better

- Respond supportively and remind her that tears for no reason are part of the menopausal process

- Ask her if there is anything you can do to help her feel better

- Ask her if she wants your company or if she would prefer to be alone

### How to Make the Situation Worse

- Tell her that if there is no reason to cry she should not be crying

- Tell her to get a "grip" and gain some self control

- Tell her you are going to leave and hopefully when you get back she will have gotten it out of her system

## Scenario 3

Your partner is on edge and looking for a fight for no reason. Nothing you do or say seems to be right.

### How to Make the Situation Better

- Do not rise to the bait; recognize that in this situation you cannot win

### How to Make the Situation Worse

- Respond defensively by stating that you have not done anything wrong

- Understand that the anger is not directed at you, and do not respond defensively

- Ask her why she is so angry. Be supportive if she says she does not know why

- Confront her anger with anger; tell her she is acting irrationally

- Tell her you think she is really losing it; suggest she seek professional help

## Scenario 4

Your partner is forgetting minor things like: signing checks, picking up prescriptions at the pharmacy, where she put her keys, etc.

| How to Make the Situation Better | How to Make the Situation Worse |
|---|---|
| • Attempt to minimize the situation; let her know it happens to everyone and it is not a sign of senile dementia | • Scold her for forgetting. |
| • Tell her that research shows that short term memory loss is symptomatic of the menopause process and will most likely reverse in time | • Suggest she contact her physician because it may be a medical condition |
| • Offer to do some of the tasks so that she has less to remember | • Simply say to her, "Let's chalk this up to old age." |

## Scenario 5

You notice while walking behind your partner that her figure has changed from youthful to matronly: gravity has taken its toll.

| How to Make the Situation Better | How to Make the Situation Worse |
|---|---|
| • When she makes comments about the changes in her body, affirm how you care for the "essence" of who she is. Tell her that everyone's body changes and you will love her at 80 as much as you did when she was 30 | • Tell her you have noticed that her body is changing, and maybe she should watch what she eats, work out more and possibly consult with a plastic surgeon |
| • Let her know that you still find her attractive, and show her that she is desirable to you | • Tell her that the aging process happens and she should get used to the way she looks |
| • Tell her that you hope her feelings about you have not changed as you know that your body has also changed and that your relationship is based upon much more than physical attractiveness | • Remind her that romance and physical attractiveness is the province of the young |

We are certain that the correct responses to the above scenarios (how to make the situation better) appear obvious to you. Were they always obvious or have they become obvious due to your increased awareness? Most likely the latter is true.

Many of us need to be reminded often of how to respond during these types of situations, which can become emotionally tense. One of the authors (who shall remain nameless) is guilty on occasion of giving a wrong response. Yes, one of the authors who wrote the book *Decoding the Enigma: His Guide to Her Menopause* (can you guess which author?). How could such a thing occur? It occurs because at times we act and react in the moment and respond defensively to words and actions without thinking. This candid admission by the author underscores the fact that unless one is truly a saint, it is difficult to be perfect, and perfection should not be the point at which the bar is set.

## WILL YOU MAKE MISTAKES? WILL YOU REGRESS?

You likely will. However what we hope has been achieved, as a result of this guide, is an awareness of the potential mistakes so that situations can be diffused before they escalate; so that you are not communicating in anger or from a sense of hurt.

## IS THERE A WAY TO COME OUT AS THE WINNER?

Remember that you are not adversaries, and there is not going to be a winner and a loser. You are in this together striving to reach a vantage point so that you can engage in mutually rewarding problem solving. You must first communicate to each other what the problem is so that it can be remedied.

Although we have provided you with examples of the words to use, strategies to make use of and clear definitions about the changes the woman in your life is going through, we know that when you are "in the moment" it still may be difficult to respond appropriately. Will incorporating all of the techniques we have provided you with in this guide make it easier for both of you to get through this stage of your lives?

The answer is: **YES**

## COMMUNICATION IS THE KEY

As we have previously indicated each of you should state your needs and points-of-view to each other. Sometimes this can be achieved face-to-face but other times it may be too emotional to communicate in person. If this is the case, consider writing a letter to your partner. What is important is that you make the attempt to convey to each other what you are feeling and what you expect from each other, so that you can arrive at a solution that each of you can support, or at least with which you can feel a sense of comfort.

## IS COMPROMISE THE ANSWER?

You may be surprised, but the answer is NO. In conflict resolution research literature, compromise is viewed as a "lose-lose" strategy. It is considered lose-lose because both parties emphasize what they gave up in the compromise rather than what they have gained.

What may be the answer, in particular if the problem is emotionally based, is to allow yourself time to cool down (give each other space) before addressing the issue. The hormonal fluctuation the menopausal woman may be experiencing can cause behavioral and/or emotional reactions that do not have a rational basis. It is difficult to address irrationality with rationality. These are the times when the most effective remedy to the situation is a simple "I understand" or if appropriate, "I'm sorry." Remember the distinction made earlier in the guide between winning battles and losing wars.

## MAYBE I SHOULD JUST SCHEDULE A LONG BUSINESS TRIP!

Six to thirteen years is an awfully long time to be away! Recall the concept of motivation we discussed earlier? Many theorists believe that if you are going to be motivated to achieve a particular task, you must first believe that you have the ability to achieve it. You have all the tools to effectively achieve the tasks, to successfully navigate through this process (and you do not have to be a saint or a shrink to be successful).

**We believe** that if **you believe** in a positive result or outcome, your relationship will not only survive but will thrive. You can never overestimate **the power of positive thinking**. Why? Because not only do you believe in yourself (part of the process of being motivated), but you also believe that your performance will lead to the results or outcomes that you value and that are positive (and avoid results and outcomes that are negative). As we have said before, you have a great deal invested in this relationship, and the fact that you have read this far in the guide is an indication that you want to make this relationship work. On the other side of the spectrum, the destruction of your relationship is an outcome that most of us would agree is psychologically and oftentimes economically negative.

## WHY IS IT GOING TO WORK?

From her shoes:

- Because it feels wonderful to know that he cares enough to understand
- How can I feel alone when I know how hard he is trying?
- Because I can still feel attractive, needed and wanted by him

From his shoes:

- Because the effort to pay attention to her needs is more important to her now than ever
- Because she still needs me (everyone needs to be needed)
- Because I have a great deal invested in this relationship, and I want to reap the benefits and make it work

## IS THAT ALL THERE IS?

In addition to the techniques we have provided to you throughout *Decoding the Enigma: His Guide to Her Menopause*, it is important that you recognize that there are many resources you can tap into to gain timely information about menopause. The Internet is one very important resource. However, when using the World Wide Web to access information, remember to choose your sources wisely. Not all information on the Web is valid. Check for evidence that the source knows about the subject matter of menopause. How can you know that?

- Check the author's credentials
    - o   Is the author an expert or an authority in the area?
- Make certain the information is up-to-date
    - o   Outdated information can be misleading
- Make certain the information is reliable
    - o   Is the information well documented?

## ON YOUR OWN...........

Remember: try your best to step into her shoes whenever possible. We know that task will not be daunting for you anymore; after all you now have a certain level of expertise because you have read *Decoding the Enigma: His Guide to Her Menopause.* We are not going to wish you "good luck" because luck is not what is needed. Instead we want to remind you that the menopausal journey does not have to be about simply surviving; you have the tools at your disposal to navigate your way so that the two of you can thrive and make this a positive experience, one that will enhance your relationship.

978-0-595-38971-1
0-595-38971-6

www.ingramcontent.com/pod-product-compliance
Lightning Source LLC
Chambersburg PA
CBHW020350290526
45785CB00005B/2222

\* 9 780595 389711 \*